The Beginner's Guide to the Mediterranean Diet

Healthy and Delectable Mediterranean Diet Recipes

By: Amy Zulpa

TABLE OF CONTENTS

Publishers Notes 3

Dedication 4

Chapter 1- What is the Mediterranean Diet? 5

Chapter 2- What Are the Benefits of the Mediterranean Diet?
.... 10

Chapter 3- What Are the Foods That Are Allowed On the Mediterranean Diet? 14

Chapter 4- 10 Mediterranean Breakfast Recipes 19

Chapter 5- 10 Mediterranean Lunch Recipes 27

Chapter 6- 10 Mediterranean Dinner Recipes 35

Chapter 7- 10 Mediterranean Dessert Recipes 43

About the Author 51

Publishers Notes

Disclaimer

This publication is intended to provide helpful and informative material. It is not intended to diagnose, treat, cure, or prevent any health problem or condition, nor is intended to replace the advice of a physician. No action should be taken solely on the contents of this book. Always consult your physician or qualified health-care professional on any matters regarding your health and before adopting any suggestions in this book or drawing inferences from it.

The author and publisher specifically disclaim all responsibility for any liability, loss or risk, personal or otherwise, which is incurred as a consequence, directly or indirectly, from the use or application of any contents of this book.

Any and all product names referenced within this book are the trademarks of their respective owners. None of these owners have sponsored, authorized, endorsed, or approved this book.

Always read all information provided by the manufacturers' product labels before using their products. The author and publisher are not responsible for claims made by manufacturers.

© 2014

Manufactured in the United States of America

DEDICATION

This book is dedicated to those who don't have a problem trying new meals.

Chapter 1 - What is the Mediterranean Diet?

Okay, just about everybody is looking for ways to stay healthy. Whether you want to lose weight, protect your heart health, lower your cholesterol, there are so many plans out there that you may not know where to start. What if I told you that there is a diet plan followed by some of the healthiest cultures in the world, and that you don't have to travel any farther than your grocery store to reap the benefits?

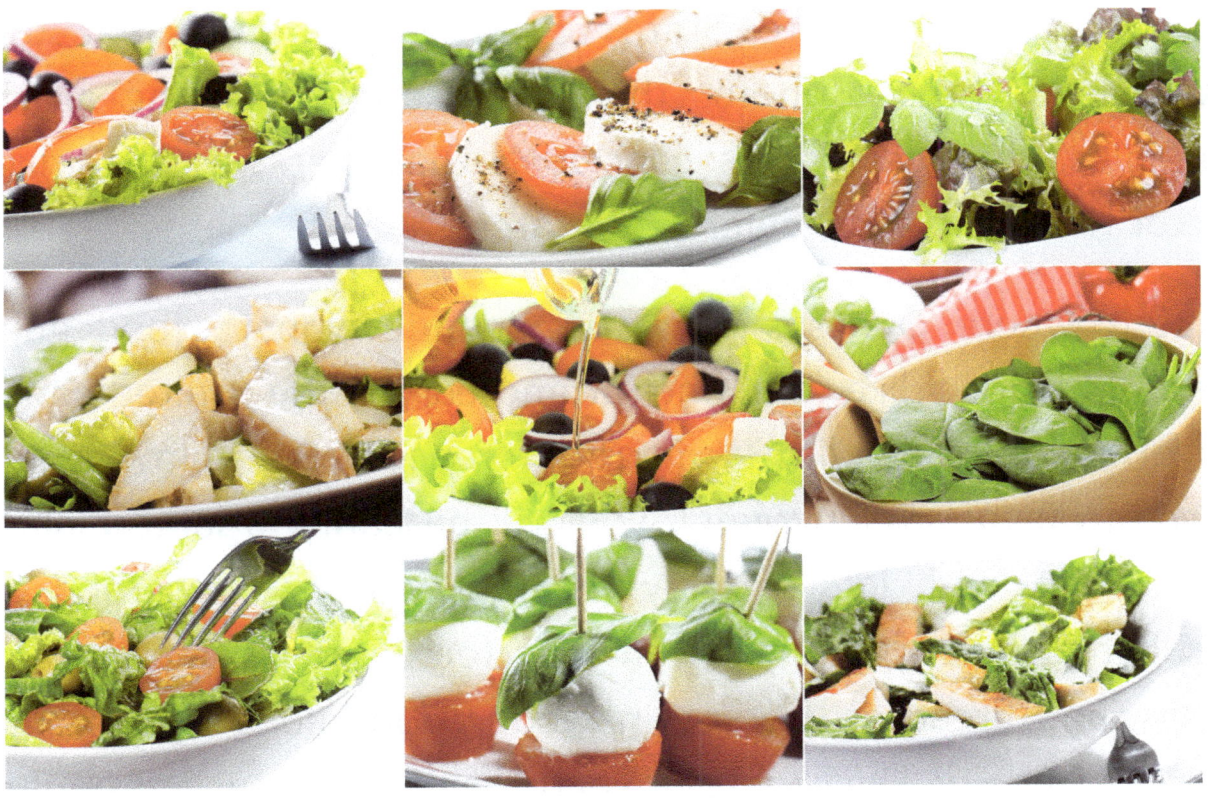

The Mediterranean diet, modeled after the traditional dining habits of people and cultures living around the Mediterranean Sea, is a set of guidelines developed by the nonprofit organization known as the Oldways Preservation and Exchange Trust, along with Harvard University School of Public Health, and the World Health Organization, in an attempt to bring Old World solutions to health and wellness to the New World problems of heart disease and obesity.

It all began with a scientific study, started in the 1940s, known as the Seven Countries Study, which examined the relationship between health and diet of people all over the world. What researchers found was that the risk of coronary death was far lower in men from the Mediterranean region than in men of the same age from the United States or Northern Europe. What could have been the reason for this? Well, after analyzing all the variables, the researchers concluded that diet was the major factor to explain such lower death rates.

That is where Oldways comes in and develops a food guide pyramid, much like the one promoted by the United States government, but with a few differences. By following the Mediterranean diet pyramid, you will be eating a largely plant-based diet, with lots of tasty vegetables, nuts, beans and oils throughout the day, and fresh fruit for dessert. Whole grains, pasta, and bread are served in moderation, along with a small amount of dairy, like cheese or yogurt, and meats such as poultry, fish, or shellfish. Wine is important to Mediterranean culture, and is incorporated into the diet for its health benefits and antioxidants. Red meat and sweets are limited to only special occasions, or a few times per month. Flavor is imparted to meals mostly by herbs and spices, instead of salt, and the best part of the Mediterranean diet is that it isn't a strict set of foods or a specific caloric count; rather, as long as you follow the general serving guidelines, you have the option to eat what you like.

With the recommendation to add more healthy oils and nuts, the Mediterranean diet pyramid is a bit higher in fat than a typical modern diet, but don't let that deter you! There is a ton of health benefits associated with the Mediterranean diet. For one, following the Mediterranean diet has been shown to lower the risk of heart disease, as well as reduce blood pressure and the bad kind of cholesterol, known as LDL cholesterol. This is a result of staying away from salt and saturated fats, like butter and lard, and including healthier monounsaturated fats and polyunsaturated fats, like olive oil and nuts. In fact, in 2013, the New England Journal of Medicine published a study which showed that up to 30 percent of strokes, heart attacks, and deaths from heart disease may be prevented by following the Mediterranean diet!

Another benefit is that the Mediterranean diet has been shown to help people lose weight. This may come from the fact that all those fibrous vegetables and fat helps the body feel fuller longer, and since the Mediterranean diet does not completely ban entire food groups, you will never feel deprived. Several studies have shown that when compared to subjects who ate a traditional low-fat diet, subjects who ate a high-fat, Mediterranean diet actually lost more weight! Since maintaining a healthy weight is essential to preventing or controlling diabetes, it is no surprise that the

Mediterranean diet could help with this goal, too. A 2013 study based on more than 22,000 participants showed that those following the Mediterranean diet most closely had a significantly lower risk of developing type 2 diabetes than those who did not follow it.

If you still don't think the Mediterranean diet is right for you, think about this: because the guidelines are so lenient on which foods are incorporated into an individual's diet, it is easily customized to meet more stringent dietary requirements. It would not be difficult to create meals that are completely vegetarian, vegan, or gluten free. If you follow religious restrictions, finding kosher or halal alternatives are also quite possible.

Now, the Mediterranean diet is more than just about food; it's about an all-around healthier lifestyle. Proponents of the diet encourage healthy activities, such as spending meal time with family and friends, enjoying and savoring your food. Also, since traditional Mediterranean people are more active than modern culture, adding activity to your life is important to promote health and weight loss. Walking, bicycle riding, even gardening or dancing are all good ways to start.

So, the next time you think it's impossible to lose those few extra pounds, or to find something healthy to eat that also tastes good, take a look at the Mediterranean diet and all it has to offer. From sliced tomatoes sprinkled with olive oil, to salmon and pasta with a glass of red wine, the possibilities are endless, and the health benefits are proven!

Chapter 2 - What Are the Benefits of the Mediterranean Diet?

The Mediterranean diet is easy to follow mainly because it gives you consistent food choices by eliminating the conflicting information people are inundated with on nearly every food product labels they see in the supermarket. Whether the Mediterranean food is low in calories or high in energy, the penchant for it by many weight-watchers has defined it all over the world.

More than two thirds of the Mediterranean dishes are based on natural ingredients, and they are easy to cook. These food choices are cheap, tasty as well as something that brings long-lasting pleasure after eating. This diet can be used on several different fronts. First, it has the benefits of a perfect weight-loss diet that have been proven to be effective for the long run. Next, it also stands on its own as a guide for a healthy lifestyle that reduces your carbon footprint. Overall, this diet can simplify your life by giving you clear choices, which is a win-win.

Mediterranean Diet is Heart Healthy

This dietary lifestyle is one of the reasons why the health-care systems in Mediterranean regions are not saddled with diabetes, heart diseases, hypertension and obesity like the western countries. In many parts of the world that follow various eating habits, Mediterranean diet is a household staple. The absence of heart conditions is a direct result of the daily food choices they make.

People who eat more plant protein tend to have lower rates of heart disease and colon cancer. What is more, people who eat more nuts and seeds have lower blood pressure and cholesterol levels than those who never eat them. The total amount of fat you eat in the form of red meat and other foods isn't really linked with heart problems. Rather, it is the type of fat that matters, and Mediterranean foods are filled with good fats. Eating enough good fat is one of the secrets of being able to stay young and stick with healthier food choices in the long run.

Mediterranean Diet Boosts Weight Loss

The Mediterranean diet is an easy and painless solution to weight woes, with people spending no more than their family budget on the products they buy to cook these foods. In contrast to most weight obsessed parts of the world where people rely on fast food on a daily basis, places where Mediterranean diet is followed is unique in that its food landscape has been shaped largely by commercial farmers and home-grown farms. Much of the cultural shift is taking place in the rest of the world because people are realizing that foods that are processed, packaged and distributed are what are causing their weight gain.

In addition, when people added 1 cup of beans and legumes a day to their diets, they lost an average of 10 pounds in the first month. So, if you are looking for real answers to your weight problems, you need to start changing your eating habits and switch to this diet. Collectively the thinking needs to be expanded beyond what is simply given on the food labels. Perhaps you are not really interested to lose weight, but you have made up your mind to eat in a reasonable way. If you are already following another diet plan with success but want to refine your existing diet, you can also simply follow this diet to see your favorite choices.

Mediterranean Diet Improves Immunity

The Mediterranean diet is not only great for the planet but great for the minds of people who eat it. All of the steps that it takes to bring those protein rich whole grains, vegetables and spices from the grocery store to your plate require will power and a small budget. And while you begin to realize the nutritional value these foods offer, the consequences of the food choices are incredible. This diet has been proven to improve immunity and prepare the body to fight against viruses and bacteria. With this diet, people are unlikely to get food allergies. Moving toward this diet means that you are embracing the kind of food that is nutrient rich.

The Mediterranean Diet is an All in One Nutrition

Now that you are following Mediterranean diet, remember that you are already getting a significant amount of vitamins and minerals. The nuts, seeds and vegetables you will be eating on this diet are going to go a long way to meet most of your nutritional needs. Need calcium without relying on dairy products? With this diet it is easy to reach your daily calcium requirement. And if you think your diet may not be high in fiber, you are wrong. This diet brings a better balance in all aspects. Following it will make you a more conscious consumer of other products.

The Mediterranean Diet Is Good For Your Pocket

Of all the diets, this Mediterranean diet is cheaper. And of all the research that has been examined, one of the consistent findings is that buying the food involved in this diet is the best strategy for saving money. If local Mediterranean food tastes better, it is no surprise that eating them can save you even more. The study also points to the positive direction when it comes to medical needs. In fact, other diets are a rich person's diet, and they are linked to diseases of affluence. All of this, in short, is why so many people are increasing the consumption of the right kinds of foods.

Chapter 3- What Are the Foods That Are Allowed On the Mediterranean Diet?

The main components of the Mediterranean diet emphasize healthy food groups such as fruits, vegetables, foods rich in protein, whole grains, beans, legumes, high-fiber, breads and nuts. The Mediterranean diet does contribute immensely to weight loss and greater health associated with reduced risk of various diseases.

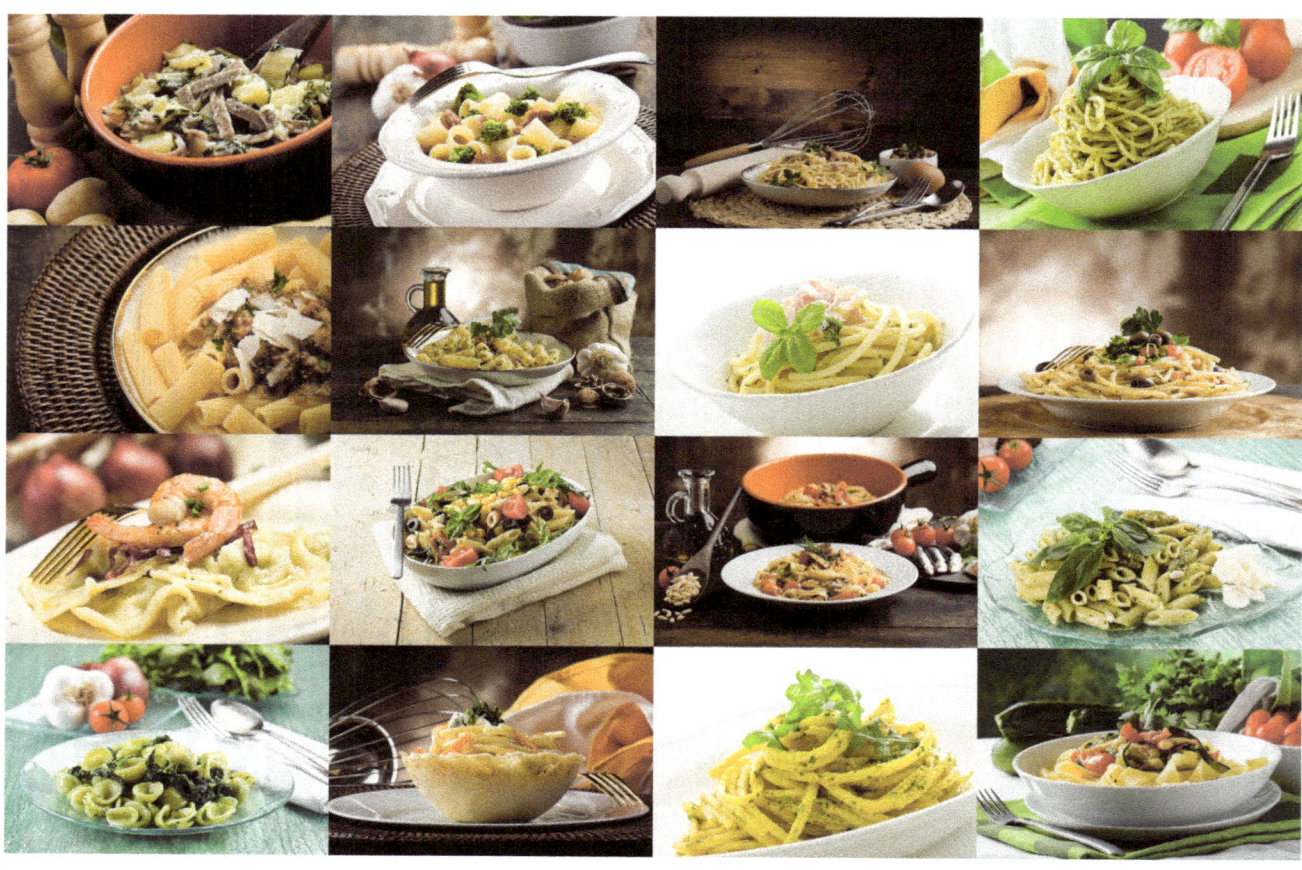

Dark leafy vegetables are foods that are also allowed on the Mediterranean diet. Broccolis are some of the green vegetables that are encouraged. Broccoli and bitter brassica and other members of the cabbage family are also included. These food types provide plenty of vitamin C, potassium, calcium and are rich in fiber. In order to add some flavor, some individuals may occasionally add anchovy, hot pepper and certain sausages. Unrefined grains which include pasta, bread, barley and couscous are the base of this diet. These grain foods provide refined versions of glucose and provide fiber, magnesium, vitamin E and antioxidants. These food groups also protect against chronic diseases. They are also known to protect against heart disease and diabetes. Beans as part of the protein group are rich in protein along with calcium, folate, iron and zinc. Chickpeas are commonly combined with grains and starches for the filling effect of fiber.

Nuts are high in amino acids, are rich sources of protein, fiber, vitamin E, folate, calcium and magnesium. Nuts are generally ground into sauces, consumed as snacks or sprinkled on salads. Hazelnuts are examples of the form of protein that are common additions to the Mediterranean diet meals. Hazelnuts are used in various recipes that include the following: Hazelnut cookies, hazelnut cakes, desert recipes, and side dishes. Chocolate Tart with Hazelnut Shortbread Crust is a popular desert and Green Beans with Bacon and hazelnut side dishes add a lot of flavor to the main course meals. For individuals that do not favor nuts, creativity in various recipes is the key.

Olive oil especially the extra virgin types are vital in Mediterranean meals especially when preparing vegetables. These oils are rich in monounsaturated fats and are also known to be rich in antioxidants. Monounsaturated fats are also known as "good" cholesterol that is essential for regular health. It has been noted that these oils explains the low rates in heart disease and lower blood pressure for those that add them in their regular meals. Precaution has to be taken when choosing these oils due to the significant difference between extra virgin olive oil and the regular oils.

Eggplants are a common addition to the Mediterranean diet. These foods are known for their flavorful texture. Eggplant comes in a variety of colors such as; purple, orange, green or striped which add a lot of color to the meals. Peppers also add color and are known to protect against macular degeneration. Pepper recipes may include bell peppers, hot peppers, and red peppers. Stuffed pepper recipes are very popular; green beans and pepper for a bell pepper side dish are favored as well. Tomatoes used for cooking or consumption comes in various forms; fresh, canned and in a form of paste. Tomatoes are rich in vitamin C, vitamin A, fiber and antioxidants. The color does contribute to the meal presentation.

Seafood is the main form of protein in this diet. Shrimp, squid, and sea bass are lean forms of seafood that provide ample protein. Although tuna may be slightly fattier, it may be added occasionally in their meals as they supply omega-3 fatty acids. Varieties of shrimp recipes do include; fried shrimp, grilled shrimp, and creamy pasta and shrimp.

Additional examples of foods that are allowed on the Mediterranean diet include the following:

- Variety of fruits and vegetables may include grapes, blueberries, spinach, olives and figs.
- Eating whole- grain foods such as oats, brown rice, and whole wheat bread, is recommended.
- Unsaturated fats may include; canola, soybean, and flaxseed.
- Saturated fats that are included are butter, coconut oil, and foods found in animal products such as meat and dairy products.
- Fish products such as tuna, salmon, herring, sardines and mackerel can be consumed twice a week.
- Low- fat dairy products such as yogurt, cheese and milk can be consumed in moderation.
- Poultry and eggs are allowed; however they ought to be consumed in moderation as in twice a week.
- Red meat these can be consumed a few times a month and these foods should be consumed in small amounts.
- Sweets and deserts can be consumed twice a week in moderation. Non sweetened drinks are to be had in moderation as well.
- Mediterranean diets do allow a glass a day of wine.

Rather than being a formal diet, the Mediterranean diet is a way of eating, it is a lifestyle change. Notably, meat cheese, and sweets are very limited. In general, the foods that are allowed are rich with fiber, omega-3 acids, fruits, vegetables, ample protein and monounsaturated fats. Mediterranean-style meals are known to lower risk of certain diseases, boost energy levels, and keep one healthy in forms of the heart, brain and any weight related issues.

The presentation of the meal does play an important role. Individuals may not care for foods such as vegetables or nuts as such the presentation and creativity may make a difference. Using herbs and spices instead of salt may be used to spruce up the flavor of the meal. It has been noted that residents of Greece average six or more servings a day of rich antioxidant-rich fruits and vegetables. These meals can be fun and enjoyable rather than referring to them as a strict diet.

Chapter 4- 10 Mediterranean Breakfast Recipes

Eating breakfast is the extremely important. That does not mean that you have to have the same old boring breakfast each morning. Spicing up your taste buds with some Mediterranean breakfast recipes will take you on a culinary journey and jump-start your day with new flavors and ingredients. These 10 Mediterranean breakfast recipes are quick and easy, and will be easy to fit into your morning breakfast routine.

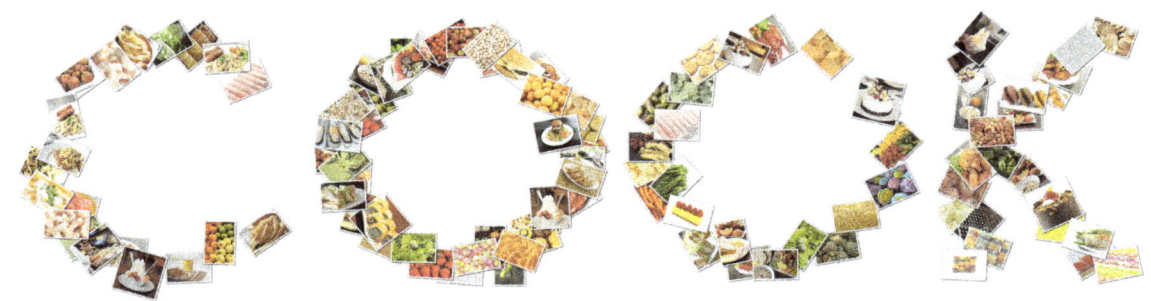

Mediterranean Yogurt Pancakes

Ingredients

1 large egg
1½ cups low-fat yogurt
¾ cup fat-free milk
1 cup whole wheat or buckwheat pancake mix

Directions

Mix yogurt, pancake mix, milk, and egg in bowl. Cook in frying pan. Top with maple syrup.

Mediterranean Breakfast Couscous

Ingredients

1 cup uncooked whole-wheat couscous
3 cups low-fat milk 1%
1 two inch cinnamon stick
6 teaspoons divided dark brown sugar
½ cup chopped dried apricots
¼ teaspoon iodized salt
4 teaspoons butter, divide and melt
¼ cup currants dried

Directions

In a pan, stir cinnamon stick and milk over heat for 3 minutes (approx. 180 degrees) medium-high.

Remove from stove, stir in currants, apricots, brown sugar, 4 teaspoons salt, and couscous. Cover and stand 15 min. Remove cinnamon stick. Divide into 4 containers and top with 1-teaspoon butter and 1/2 teaspoon brown sugar. Serve hot.

Mediterranean Muesli

Ingredients

1 cup oats regular
1 cup low-fat yogurt plain
1 cup low-fat milk 1%

½ cup walnuts chopped coarsely

⅓ cup honey

¼ cup oat bran

3 tablespoons dried chopped apricots

3 tablespoons dried chopped figs

3 tablespoons pitted chopped dates

Optional raspberries or other fresh berries

Directions

Combine all ingredients except berries in bowl. Refrigerate for 2 hours then garnish with fresh berries if wanted.

Mediterranean Bagel Snacks

Ingredients

2 slices red onion

2 tablespoons hummus roasted garlic flavored

2 plain bagels, toasted and split

2 tablespoons cut into strips drained jar roasted red peppers

4 slices deli roast beef thin

½ cup baby arugula water packed leaves chopped

Directions

On each half of bagel, spread 1 ½ teaspoons hummus. Divide the pepper strips, beef, arugula, and onion on bagel halves. Place tops on halves of bagels

Cut each bagel into bite-sized pieces and skewer with toothpicks.

Mediterranean Breakfast Quinoa

Ingredients

1 teaspoon sea salt
2 cups milk
¼ cup chopped almonds
1 teaspoon cinnamon ground
1 cup quinoa
2 finely diced dried pitted dates
1 teaspoon vanilla extract
2 tablespoons honey
5 dried apricots, finely chopped

Directions

Brown almonds over medium heat, 3-5 minutes and reserve.

Heat quinoa and cinnamon until warm. Stir in salt and milk. Heat to boil and then reduce heat to low, cover and let simmer for 15 minutes. Stir dates, vanilla, apricots, honey, and 1/2 almonds in. Sprinkle with remaining almonds.

Greek Baba Ganoush Recipe

Ingredients

1 large roasted, peeled, chopped eggplant
2 tablespoons tahini

½ tablespoon lemon juice

3 tablespoons extra virgin olive oil

1 large crushed garlic clove

¼ cup (4 tbsp) low fat plain yogurt

1 pinch salt

1 dash pepper

1 tablespoon chopped parsley

Directions

Warm the oven to 400 degrees. On flat sheet, cook eggplant for 20 minutes per each side. Cool, peel and cut.

In a blender mix the garlic, eggplant, tahini, plain yogurt, lemon juice, salt, olive oil, and black pepper. The mixture should be creamy; if over thick add oil or water.

Pour the mixture out of the blender onto a serving plate. Top with sprinkle of oil and parsley. Offer with pita bread.

Cheesy Mediterranean Scramble

Ingredients

3 cartons egg substitute (4 oz each)

⅛ teaspoon black pepper ground

1 12 tablespoons butter or margarine

½ teaspoon dried crushed basil leaves

6 slices whole wheat bread toast

1 finely chopped small red bell pepper

2 tablespoon crumbled feta cheese
1 finely chopped small sweet onion

Directions

Beat then set aside egg substitute, black pepper, and basil with fork.

In skillet, melt butter over medium-high heat. Add red pepper and onion 4 minutes. Add egg mixture. After a few minutes, stir periodically until cooked, and set. Add cheese to top and serve with toast.

Egg-Crust Vegetarian Breakfast Pizza

Ingredients

3 teaspoons olive oil
4 oz thick sliced and washed mushrooms 6 sliced black olives
¼ green pepper sliced thinly
1 oz low fat mozzarella
2 eggs well beaten
½ teaspoon seasoning to taste (spike)
¼ teaspoon to taste dried oregano

Directions

Brown the mushrooms in a little oil. Remove from pan. Add little more oil to frying pan, heat and add eggs, oregano, and seasoning.

When eggs are 1/2 cooked layer mushrooms, cheese, and peppers. Cook covered for 3-4 minutes. Remove cover and place under broiler for 2-4 minutes.

Mediterranean Scramble

Ingredients

1 tablespoon heavy cream, milk, or half & half
2 eggs
Butter
¼ cup chopped spinach
2 tablespoons diced zucchini
2 tablespoons crumbled feta
Salt
Fresh ground pepper

Directions

In bowl mix milk and eggs. Heat pan over medium-low heat. Add butter to cover pan and add eggs.

When eggs start to harden, use utensil to move eggs from outside to middle of pan. As eggs form curds add spinach, feta, and zucchini stirring until set.

Paprika Eggs

Ingredients

4 eggs sliced hard boiled

1 teaspoon olive oil

½ teaspoon paprika

½ teaspoon salt, kosher

Directions

Coat olive oil on egg slices. Season with pepper, salt, and paprika.

Chapter 5- 10 Mediterranean Lunch Recipes

Shrimp & Spicy Tomatoes

Ingredients

2 large carrots, chopped
8 oz. green beans, ½ inch pieces
1 cup whole wheat Israeli couscous
1 tablespoon olive oil
1 large onion, chopped
1 can (14.5 oz.) fire-roasted diced tomatoes, un-drained
1 pound shrimp, peeled, deveined

Directions

In a large microwave-safe bowl, combine carrots, green beans, and 1 tablespoon water. Cover with vented plastic top. Microwave for 5 minutes, or until just tender.

Meanwhile, prepare couscous as per instructions on package.

In a skillet, heat oil on medium-high. Add onion; cook 5 minutes or until golden, stirring. Add carrot mixture and tomatoes. Heat to boiling, reduce heat to medium. Add shrimp; cook 5 minutes, stirring occasionally. Serve over couscous.

Grilled Eggplant Roll-Ups

Ingredients

4 medium eggplants, sliced ¼" thick
3 tablespoons plus ¼ cup olive oil, divided
2 cups crumbled feta cheese
1 jalapeno, seeded and minced
1 tablespoon fresh lemon juice
3 tablespoon chopped fresh mint, divided

Directions

Heat gas grill to medium-high. Set eggplant on rack; brush with 3 tablespoons olive oil. Grill 4-5 minutes, turning once. Mash together feta, ¼ cup oil, jalapeno, lemon juice and 1 tablespoon mint. Evenly divide feta mixture over eggplant slices and roll up. Sprinkle with rest of mint.

Mediterranean Broccoli Rabe

Ingredients

½ cup plus 4 tablespoons olive oil, divided
4 large cloves garlic, sliced
1 teaspoon red pepper flakes
4 bunches broccoli rabe, trimmed, blanched, divided
¼ cup golden raisins, divided
¼ cup Pignoli nuts, toasted, divided
Salt
Pepper

Directions

Heat ½ cup olive oil, garlic and red pepper flakes in skillet over medium-low heat for 10 minutes, until garlic is slightly browned; set aside. Working in batches, in large skillet heat 2 Tablespoons oil over medium-high heat. Add half the broccoli rabe. Sauté until heated through. Toss with half the raisins, nuts and seasoned oil. Repeat with other ingredients. Toss; salt and pepper to taste.

Marinated Lemon Chicken

Ingredients

Marinade and chicken
3 garlic cloves minced
1 tablespoon olive oil
1 tablespoon sugar
1 tablespoon chopped fresh rosemary
2 teaspoon fresh thyme
2 teaspoon finely grated lemon rind
Salt and pepper to taste
4 bone-in chicken breasts

Basting Sauce

½ cup fresh lemon juice
2 tablespoon olive oil
1 tablespoon red wine vinegar
2 teaspoons honey mustard

Directions

For marinade, combine first 7 ingredients in large bowl. Add chicken, toss until well-coated. Cover, refrigerate overnight.

For basting sauce, combine all ingredients in medium bowl, whisk.

Place chicken on pre-heated grill rack. Grill 16 minutes, turning once. Baste chicken with lemon-juice mixture. Grill about 8 more minutes, until done.

Veggie Ceviche

Ingredients

1 can (14 oz.) artichoke hearts, drained, chopped
1 large tomato, chopped
¼ pound white mushrooms, chopped
⅓ cup chopped scallions
1 large garlic clove, minced
¼ cup fresh lime juice
¼ cup olive oil
1 ripe avocado, peeled, pitted, chopped
Salt and pepper
Whole wheat pita wedges

Directions

In medium bowl, combine first 7 ingredients. Cover with plastic wrap and refrigerate 30-minutes. Stir in avocado; season with salt and pepper. Serve with pita wedges.

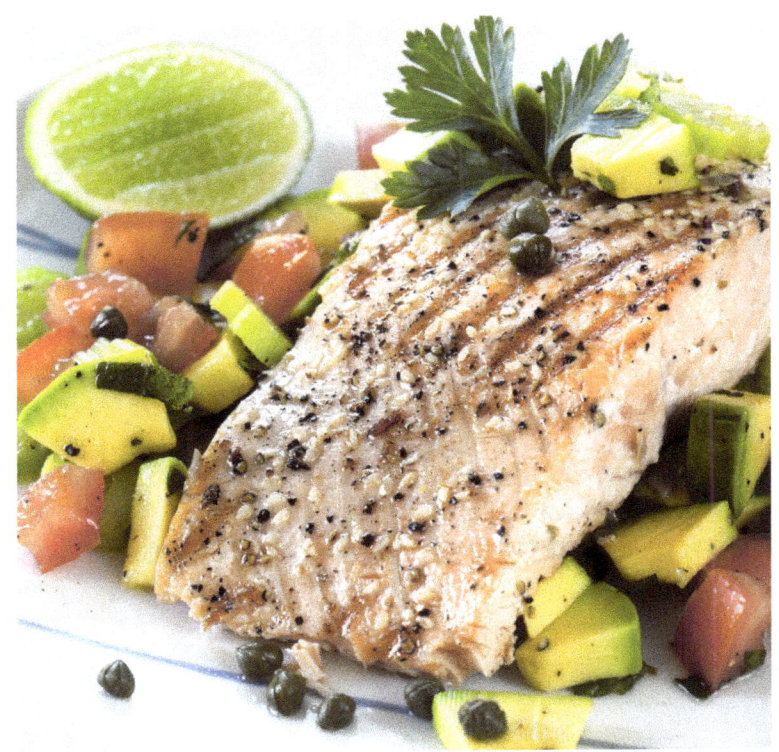

Salmon Mediterranean Style

Ingredients

Salt and pepper to season
4 skinless salmon fillets
Cooking spray
2 large tomatoes, chopped
½ cup chopped zucchini
2 tablespoon capers (not drained)
1 tablespoon olive oil
3 oz. kalamata olives, sliced

Directions

Preheat oven to 425 degrees Fahrenheit.

Sprinkle salt and pepper over salmon. Place salmon in an 11 x 7 baking dish coated with cooking spray. Combine tomatoes and remaining ingredients in a bowl; spoon mixture over salmon. Bake for 22 minutes.

Salmon Burgers

Ingredients

1 lb. skinless salmon fillets cut into 2-inch pieces
1/2 c breadcrumbs
1 lg egg white
1 pinch salt
1/4 teaspoon black pepper
1/2 c cucumber slices
1/4 c crumbled feta cheese
4 ciabatta rolls, toasted

Directions

In a food processor, pulse salmon, panko, and egg white until salmon finely chopped.

Form into 4 patties; Add salt and pepper.

Heat the grill to medium-high and let cook, turn once, until burgers are just cooked through, about 7 minutes per side. Serve with buns.

Mediterranean Chicken Salad

Ingredients

3 grilled chicken breasts, chopped
1 (15 oz.) can chickpeas rinsed, drained
1 cup chopped cucumber
½ cup chopped green onion
¼ cup chopped fresh mint
½ cup plain yogurt
2 garlic cloves, minced
¼ teaspoon salt
2 cup baby spinach leaves
⅓ cup feta cheese
Lemon wedges

Directions

Combine first 8 ingredients; toss gently. Fold in spinach and feta. Serve with lemon wedges.

Peasant Salad

Ingredients

3 tomatoes, chopped
1 cucumber, diced
1 small red onion, sliced
½ cup kalamata olives
½ cup olive oil
½ pound feta cheese, crumbled

1 tablespoon chopped fresh oregano
Salt and pepper

Directions

In a bowl, combine tomatoes, cucumber, onion and olives. Drizzle with olive oil. Sprinkle with feta and oregano. Salt and pepper to taste.

Halibut Greek-Style

Ingredients

4 halibut fillets
1 onion, chopped
5 oz. kalamata olives
¼ cup capers
¼ cup olive oil
1 tablespoon lemon juice
Salt and pepper

Directions

Preheat oven to 350 degrees Fahrenheit. Place halibut on a large sheet of aluminum foil.

Combine remaining ingredients in a bowl. Spoon tomato mixture over halibut. Seal all edges of foil. Place packet on baking sheet.

Bake until fish flakes easily, 30-40 minutes.

Chapter 6- 10 Mediterranean Dinner Recipes

The Mediterranean diet emphasizes dishes made with vegetables, legumes, whole grains and olive oil. As mentioned throughout this book, fruit is also a large component of a Mediterranean based diet. Most protein comes in the form of fish, and poultry, red meat and cheese are to be eaten sparingly. Often people become tired of limiting their intake of certain foods in order to stick to a Mediterranean type diet. The reality is, with the addition of herbs and citrus you can have a varied and tasty diet that stays well within the Mediterranean diet guidelines.

Seared Tuna Steaks

Ingredients

Ahi Tuna Steaks
1 tablespoon lemon juice
1 tablespoon soy sauce
1 clove crushed garlic
1 tablespoon olive oil

Directions

Combine lemon juice, soy sauce and crushed garlic in a bowl. Marinate the tuna steaks while bringing a sauté or grill pan to medium high heat. Add the olive to sauté pan or coat carefully coat the grill pan. Sear the tuna steaks for 1 minute on each side leaving the tuna extremely rare in the middle and creating a crust on the outside of the fish.

Serve with salad or lentils.

Lentils with Shallots and Carrots

Ingredients

1 cup green lentils (often available in the bulk aisle)
2 cups water or vegetable stock
1 large shallot, finely minced
1 large carrot finely diced
1 tablespoon olive oil

Directions

Heat olive oil on medium heat. Add the shallot and carrot and sauté until slightly tender. About five minutes. Add water or stock and bring to a rapid simmer. Rinse the lentils then add them to the pot. Simmer twenty to thirty minutes uncovered until lentils are tender. Add water or stock as needed. Season with salt and pepper before serving.

Greek Salad

Ingredients

1 red onion finely sliced
1-2 cucumbers sliced into rounds
1-2 tomatoes sliced in to wedges

2 oz. feta cheese

1 handful black kalamata olives

¼ cup olive oil

3 tablespoon red wine vinegar

Directions

Whisk olive oil and vinegar together in a large bowl. Add vegetables and toss. Before serving crumble the feta over the salad and toss again.

Most dinner recipes can easily be eaten for lunch but here are a few that work well on the go.

Chopped Salad with Tuna and Oregano Dressing

Ingredients

2-3 cups chopped salad greens
1 can of quality water packed tuna, drained
1 cucumber, roughly chopped
1 red bell pepper, roughly chopped
½ red onion roughly chopped

For the Dressing

½ cup olive oil

3 tablespoon red wine vinegar

1 tablespoon lemon juice

1 teaspoon oregano

Directions

Combine ingredients for dressing and allow the flavors to develop. Add salad greens and chopped vegetables to a bowl. Dress lightly with the dressing. Top with tuna and drizzle more dressing over the top of the dish before serving.

Whole Grain Pita's Stuffed With Greek Tuna Salad

Ingredients

1 whole grain pita, slice into two halves
1 can quality water packed tuna
¼ chopped celery
1 handful of kalamata olives, chopped
1 drizzle of olive oil
1 teaspoon chopped dill
Salt and pepper to taste

Directions

Combine all ingredients except for the pita. Allow to sit for 15 minutes. Stuff the pita's with the tuna mixture. This also makes a great on the go lunch.

Mediterranean "Burgers"

Ingredients

One package ground chicken (roughly one pound)
½ diced red onion

1 tablespoon dill, divided

1 egg

1 container of plain Greek yogurt

½ cucumber, grated

1 tablespoon lemon juice

2 whole grain pitas

Directions

Combine yogurt, ½ of the dill, the grated cucumber and lemon juice in a bowl. Refrigerate. Next, combine the remaining ingredients, except the pitas, and form into four burger patties. Grill or pan fry the burgers until done. Insert the burgers into the pitas and top with yogurt sauce.

Pan Seared Salmon with Roasted Mediterranean Vegetables

This is the simplest of recipes.

Ingredients

Several filets of salmon

Olive oil

Salt

Pepper

1 red onion, roughly chopped

2 zucchini, sliced

1-2 red or yellow bell peppers, roughly chopped

Cherry tomatoes, left whole

Directions

This is definitely the easiest recipe ever. Toss vegetables with olive oil, salt and pepper. Roast in a 400 degree oven 15-20. Depending on how roasted you like your vegetables.

Heat olive oil in a pan on medium heat. Salt and pepper the salmon. Pan fry until internal temperature of salmon reaches 140.

Orzo Salad

Orzo is rice shaped pasta that can be found near the spaghetti.

Ingredients

2 cups orzo cooked according to package directions
6-7 cherry tomatoes, sliced in half
4 oz. feta cheese, crumbled
Dill to taste
¼ cup olive oil
1 tablespoon balsamic oil
Salt and pepper to taste

Directions

Combine olive oil and balsamic. Combine the rest of the ingredients in a large bowl. Dress the rest of the ingredients with the dressing. Allow the salad to sit at room temperature for ten to fifteen minutes so flavors develop.

Warm Whole Grain Cereal

It's not just for breakfast! As a matter of fact people all over the world, not just people in the Mediterranean regions, eat some form of this for dinner all the time. It's filling and extremely healthy. Just make your favorite warm cereal: oatmeal, cream of wheat, whatever you prefer. You can play with the toppings and add just about anything. You can sweeten it by adding honey and fruit. It is also great with the addition of chopped dried fruit and nuts.

Artichoke, Pepper and Tuna Salad

Ingredients

16 whole wheat crackers (reduced-fat)
1 jar chopped roasted red bell peppers (drained)
2 cans albacore tuna in water (drain then flake)
2 cups fresh baby spinach leaves (chopped)
2 cloves finely chopped garlic
½ teaspoon pepper (freshly ground)
1 tablespoon lemon juice (fresh)
1 tablespoon extra-virgin olive oil
¼ cup fresh dill weed (chopped)
2 jars artichoke hearts (marinated)

Directions

Drain the artichokes and chop them up. Keep two tablespoons of the marinade for later on.

In a big bowl mix the garlic, pepper, lemon juice, oil, dill, reserved marinade and artichokes. Put in the roasted peppers, tuna and spinach and toss to combine. Serve with crackers.

Chapter 7- 10 Mediterranean Dessert Recipes

Baked Cinnamon Quince

Ingredients

3 quince, unpeeled, halved, washed and cored
18 whole cloves
1½ cups water
½ cup port wine
3 cinnamon sticks
⅓ cup white sugar

Directions

Preheat oven to 375 degrees.

Place three cloves into each half of quince. Place the quince cut-side down in a roasting pan. Add wine, water, and cinnamon sticks in the pan. Sprinkle sugar over the quince.

Bake for 35 minutes. Turn the quince over and bake for 10 minutes. Remove the pan from the oven and let the quince cool.

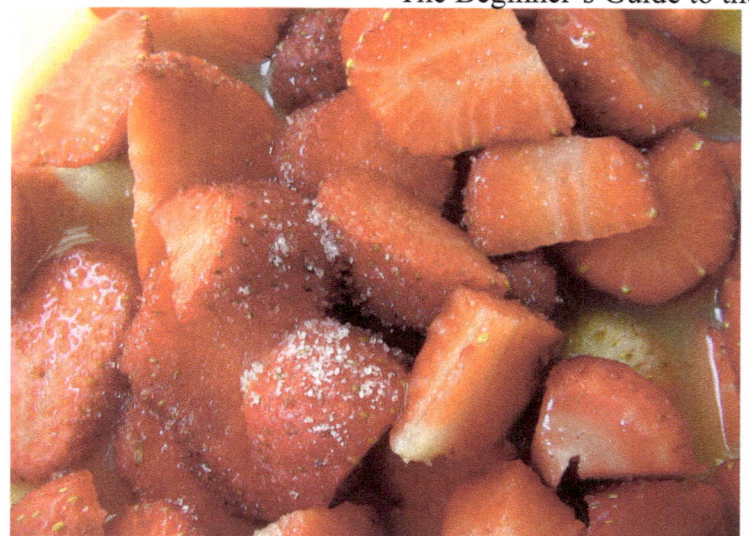

Cannoli

Ingredients

2 cups ricotta cheese

⅓ cup powdered sugar

1 teaspoon vanilla extract

2 tablespoon grated orange peel

4 tablespoon mini chocolate chips

12 small cannoli shells

¼ cup pistachios, finely chopped

Directions

Combine ricotta and powdered sugar in a bowl. Mix until creamy. Stir in vanilla, orange peel, and chocolate chips.

Fill cannoli shells with ricotta mixture. Sprinkle ends of cannoli with pistachios, sprinkle powdered sugar over each cannoli.

Holiday Cookies (Kourabiéthes)

Ingredients

2 sticks butter

½ cup powdered sugar

2 teaspoon vanilla extract

1 tablespoon milk

1 egg

2¼ cups flour

¼ teaspoon baking powder

¼ teaspoon salt

¾ cup slivered almonds

Directions

Preheat oven to 350 degrees Fahrenheit. Combine butter and powdered sugar in a bowl. Mix for about 5 minutes, until fluffy.

Add vanilla extract, milk, and egg. Mix well. Sift flour, baking powder, and salt over egg mixture. Beat well until thoroughly blended. Stir in toasted almonds.

Scoop up 1 to 2 teaspoons of dough. Use your hands to form it into a ball, crescent, or S-shape. Place on baking sheet. Bake 20 minutes, or until light golden brown.

Let cool for 15 minutes. Roll cookies in sugar.

Couscous with Butter

Ingredients

2¼ cup water

¼ teaspoon salt

2 cups couscous

1 tablespoon oil

⅓ cup raisins

3 tablespoons butter

2½ tablespoon sugar

Directions

Bring water and salt to a boil. Remove from heat, stir in couscous. Cover and let sit for 5 minutes. Add oil and mix with a fork.

Heat a few cups of water over medium heat. Place couscous in the pot to steam. Add raisins. Mix well, steam 10 minutes longer.

Add butter to couscous. Pour couscous onto a platter. Form couscous into a rough cone shape and sprinkle sugar over all.

Cheese and Melon

Ingredients

2 tablespoons olive oil

8 ounces halloumi cheese

4 slices watermelon

6 pieces pita bread

Directions

Place olive oil in medium skillet. Heat over medium flame. Add halloumi slices. Cook until lightly browned.

Arrange halloumi slices, watermelon slices, and pita bread on platter and serve.

Baklava

Ingredients

1 pound chopped mixed nuts
1 teaspoon cinnamon
1 package phyllo dough
1 cup butter
½ cup honey
1 teaspoon vanilla extract
1 teaspoon grated lemon zest
1 cup white sugar
1 cup water

Directions

Preheat to 350 degrees Fahrenheit. Butter baking dish.

Mix cinnamon and nuts. Cut dough in half to fit the dish.

Place two sheets of dough in the baking dish. Brush with butter. Add sprinkles of nut mixture. Repeat layers until all ingredients are used, ending with about 6 sheets of dough. Cut baklava into four rows, then cut diagonally to make 36 pieces. Bake 50 minutes.

Combine water and sugar in small saucepan. Bring to a boil. Stir in vanilla, honey, and lemon zest. Let it simmer for 20 minutes.

Once ready, spoon the syrup over baklava. Cool before serving.

Vasilopita

Ingredients

1 cup butter
2 cups white sugar
5 eggs
2 tablespoons water
2 teaspoons vanilla extract
3 cups flour
1 teaspoon baking powder
½ cup slivered almonds
2 tablespoons sesame seeds

Directions

Preheat oven to 325 degrees Fahrenheit. Mix butter and sugar in a bowl. Add 2 egg yolks. Stir in vanilla and water.

In another bowl, mix baking powder and flour. Add to the creamed mixture. Whip 3 egg whites. Add 1 tablespoon sugar. Mix whites into batter.

Pour batter into greased tube pan. Sprinkle seeds and nuts on the batter. Bake 70 minutes.

Greek Lemon Cake

Ingredients

3 cups flour
1 teaspoon baking soda
¼ teaspoon salt
6 eggs
2 cups white sugar
1 cup butter
2 teaspoons grated lemon zest
2 tablespoons lemon juice
1 cup plain yogurt

Directions

Preheat oven to 350 degrees Fahrenheit. Grease 10 inch tube pan. Sift baking soda, flour, and salt. Set aside. Beat egg whites in a bowl. Add ½ cup of sugar. Set aside.

Cream the butter, lemon zest, lemon juice, egg yolks and sugar together. Gently add in the other two mixtures.

Bake at 350 degrees for 60 minutes.

Semolina Pudding

Ingredients

1 cup water
1½ cups milk
1½ cups white sugar
1 cinnamon stick
½ cup butter
1 cup semolina flour

Directions

Place milk, cinnamon, sugar and water in saucepan over medium heat. Bring it to a boil. Remove cinnamon.

Melt butter in another pan. Stir in semolina until mixture is smooth and brown. Stir in the milk mixture. Stir until thick. Place in a dish. Serve warm or cold.

Frozen Greek Yogurt

Ingredients

3 cups plain whole-milk Greek yogurt
1 tablespoon lemon juice
5 tablespoons honey
10 chopped fresh mint leaves

Directions

Stir together lemon juice and yogurt until smooth.

In a separate bowl, combine mint and honey. Pour honey on top of the yogurt. Stir just a bit. Freeze for 1 to 2 hours.

ABOUT THE AUTHOR

Amy Zulpa has a great love for food and is willing to try new healthy recipes as she learns about them. Though the Mediterranean diet is not a new phenomenon, it is not something that she has tried before.

As an individual that fully believes in promoting anything that she finds helpful like a healthy recipe or a new form of exercise, she chose to write a book to introduce the non-informed readers about the benefits of the Mediterranean recipes and also to supply the reader with a few recipes that they could try to see if the diet was for them.

www.ingramcontent.com/pod-product-compliance
Ingram Content Group UK Ltd.
Pitfield, Milton Keynes, MK11 3LW, UK
UKHW050419240426
12048UKWH00014B/711